Plants As Medicine

Vol.1 Pain, Inflammation, And Gout

Written by Lawrence Pate III

In Association with Papa Bear's Pantry

Table of Contents

(*) Means refer to Glossary at the end of book for definition or process

PREFACE

Healing the root of a condition and not just the symptoms, are rarely as easy as just consuming a pill or a plant. Most healing requires a lifestyle change, and a consistent commitment to rid our bodies and minds of the readily available toxins we consume and exist around. As silly as it sounds, some physical issues are the result of our responses to negative external conditions, and changing that environment, or how we respond to that environment, usually fixes the problem.

Here is an example; stress causes our bodies to leech or lose Vitamin C. The rapid loss of Vitamin C can cause us to become more susceptible to infection, illness, and disease. Orange juice is a great go-to for a cold, but for adults, confronting the issue that is causing the stress, and finding a positive way to de-stress regularly, is just as powerful as any herbal remedy.

Healing has a lot to do with faith and belief; belief that the cure will work, and faith that you will get better and not worse. The body follows where the mind leads, and the mind is driven to where your focus demands it to go. To be healed, one must first believe that they can be healed, before the medicine is even taken.

Disclaimer:

The information and recipes presented in this book are not intended to diagnose any medical conditions. Of course, by law we cannot guarantee or claim a cure to anything, and that's why we don't claim or guarantee any type of cure for anything. It is always best to check with your doctor first concerning any medical issues, let them diagnose you, then explore natural alternatives to synthetic medications. Author assumes no liability.

Recipe 1: Cayenne Pepper Oil

(Topical)

You will need:

1/2 cup of Olive oil

3 tbsp. of Cayenne Pepper

3 tbsp. of Ginger Powder

Mason Jar

Crock-pot

(optional: 4 extra strength add ½ cup Comfrey Root)

Directions:

-Put ingredients in Mason Jar.

-Infuse in crock-pot overnight. (*Directions on infusing in glossary)

-Apply as needed generously to areas of pain.

Note:

When applying Cayenne Pepper Oil, keep hands out of eyes, ears, mouth, and private areas!

Recipe 2: Cayenne Pepper Tea

(Relieves migraine headaches.)

You will need:

¼ tsp. to 1 tbsp. of Cayenne (or as much you can handle)

1/2 lemon juice

8 oz. of purified water

Honey or Maple syrup to taste

Directions:

-Mix ingredients together and consume every 6 hrs. or as needed for pain.

 *Note: Drink Cayenne Pepper Tea and rub Cayenne Pepper Oil regularly. Your body will build up a pain guard for future pain.

Recipe 3: Raspberry Willow Bark Tea

You will need:

1 to 2 tsp. of Willow Bark

1 Raspberry tea bag or 1 tsp. of ground Raspberry Leaf

8 - 12 oz. purified of water

Honey, sugar, or maple syrup to taste

Directions:

-Put ingredients in pot, boil for 15 mins. Remove from heat and drink.

-Consume every 5 hrs. as needed for pain.

-To sweeten I use a 2:1 honey, organic sugar ratio, or just honey to taste.

*Note: DO NOT take Willow Bark with other pain medications or blood thinners.

Recipe 4: Inflammation Tonic Recipe

You will need:

2 cups of purified water

1 Raspberry tea bag (1 tsp.)

1 tbsp. Turmeric Root or powder

1 tsp. Ginger Root or powder

Honey and or sugar to taste

(Optional) 1 cup Orange Juice (Optional for diabetics)

Directions:

-Add ingredients to pot

-Boil for 10 mins

-2:1 ratio organic honey: organic sugar

(Optional) -Can add 1 cup Orange Juice (Optional for diabetics)

-Drink every 4 hrs. as needed.

Recipe 5: Pain Relief Salve

(Topical)

You will need:

1 tbsp. Chickweed Powder

1 tbsp. Wormwood Powder

10 drops Tea Tree oil

4 cups of Sweet Olive Oil

3 oz. Beeswax

Cheese Cloth

2 Mason Jars

Directions:

-Put Beeswax, chickweed, wormwood, and Sweet Olive Oil in a Mason Jar and *infuse overnight.

-Strain through cheese cloth into different clean glass jar.

-Once strained add Tea Tree Oil. Keep in Cool dry place. Apply to area as needed for pain.

Recipe 6: Pain Foot Cream

(Topical)

You will need:

10 oz. Coconut Oil (solid, not fractionated)

2 oz. Jojoba Oil

3 oz. Olive Oil

3 tbs. Candelilla Wax

1/2 oz. Beeswax

1 oz. Cocoa Butter

.5 oz. Menthol Crystals (Strong, may need a mask when adding.)

10 drops Peppermint Essential Oil

10 drops Eucalyptus Essential Oil

10 drops Niaouli Essential Oil

Directions:

-Melt all ingredients together except for the Menthol and Essential Oils.

-Remove from heat, stir in Menthol Crystals, re-heat until crystals are melted if needed.

-Remove from heat and let cool before stirring in the Essential Oils or they will evaporate, pour into containers.

-Apply as needed to areas of pain.

Recipe 7: Turmeric Pain Rub

(Topical)

You will need:

5 tbsp. Mustard Seed Oil or Sesame Seed Oil

2 tbsp. Turmeric Powder

2 tbsp. Chili Powder

1 tbsp. Neem Powder

2 tbsp. Ginger Powder

2 tbsp. Beeswax

Directions:

-Put all ingredients in Mason Jar and *infuse overnight.

-Use cheese cloth to strain. Store in dark container.

-Apply to areas of pain and use as needed.

*Note: Be advised that Turmeric will stain anything it touches, for a few days.

Recipe 8: 2 Quick Pain Relief Oil Mixes

(Topical)

Oil 1)

You will need:

2 tsp. Cayenne Pepper

1 tsp. Ginger powder

10 drops Peppermint Essential Oil

1 tb. Olive Oil

Directions:

In a small Mason Jar combine above ingredients, shake jar to mix and use as needed.

Oil 2)

In a small Mason Jar combine:

2 tsp. Cayenne Pepper

10 drops Wintergreen essential oil.

1 tb Olive Oil

Shake well in jar and use as needed.

Note: When applying, DO NOT rub eyes, nose, or mouth.

Recipe 9: Tonic 7

(4 Arthritis/Inflammation)

You will need:

6 cups of fresh Orange Juice or water

1 tsp. Cinnamon Powder

¼ tsp. Ginger Powder

1 bag Tangerine Tea

½ cup Braggs Apple Cider Vinegar

¼ tsp 90k H.U. Cayenne Pepper

½ cup raw honey

3 tbsp 10ppm Colloidal Silver

(Add silver after tonic is strained)

Cheese cloth

Directions:

-Combine all ingredients in large container.

-Steep overnight in fridge and strain through cheese cloth.

-Add Colloidal Silver now.

-Consume as much as you want.

-Will keep in fridge for at least 30 days with Colloidal Silver added.

-Make new batch for tomorrow.

-For best results take Tonic 7 daily.

Along with Tonic 7, as an Anti-Arthritis/Inflammation regiment consume:

1 tbsp. Turmeric twice a day

2 tbsp. of Powder Beef Gelatin or Chicken Bone Broth

Eat lots of Broccoli and Spinach

Should see results after 7 days.

Recipe 10: Clove Oil for Tooth Pain

(Oral)

You will need:

Clove essential oil Sesame seed oil Cotton ball

Directions:

-Dilute 2 to 3 drops Clove Oil in 1/4 tsp. of Sesame Seed Oil

-Put mixture on a cotton ball and dab affected area.

-Repeat as needed, every night

Recipe 11: Electric Daisy

This plant goes by many names, Jamba, Electric Daisy, Buzz Buttons, Para Cress, & Acmella Oleracea's leaves.

-Can chew on the flower heads (yellow and red pods) and will relieve pain and tooth pain.

-Can also be *infused in Safflower Oil and applied topically.

Recipe 12: Pineapple Pepper Drink

(For pain and inflammation)

You will need:

Inner white rind from a citrus fruit (Grapefruit or Pomelo fruit.)

1 tsp. Cayenne

1 tsp. Hot Paprika

1 tsp. Turmeric

1 cup water

1 whole Pineapple

(Optional: MSM supplements and B1 Vitamins for added anti-pain support).

Directions:

-In a blender break up white inner rind of citrus fruit.

-Add 1 tbsp of: Cayenne, Hot Paprika, and Turmeric.

-Add 1 cup distilled water (more water less strength).

-Cut outer pineapple (skin) off.

-Chop the rest of the pineapple and add to blender.

-Blend well and drink 8 to 12 oz. every 5 hrs. or as needed for pain.

(Optional)

-Take daily with MSM and B1 Vitamins for added anti-pain support.

-This is a daily tonic so if you are taking blood thinners, take medications and this tea 4hrs apart. This can potentially replace blood thinners.

Recipe 13: Anti-Pain Oil

(Topical)

You will need:

2 tbsp. Pure Aloe

2 tbsp. Emu oil

1 tbsp. MSM Powder

1 tbsp. Vit E

10 drops of Peppermint Essential Oil

15 drops of Frankincense Essential Oil

15 drops of Myrrh Essential Oil

15 drops of Eucalyptus Essential Oil

15 drops of Clove Essential Oil

15 drops Black Pepper Essential Oil

1 tbsp. Colloidal Silver Gel (optional)

Directions:

In a glass bowl or jar combine all ingredients.

Mix well. Apply to pain area: base of spin, top of feet, base of neck, or behind knees.

Can apply by hands or put in roll-on container.

Recipe 14: Wild Lettuce (Opium Lettuce) Pain Killer

Wild Lettuce is unscheduled by the FDA and is legal to grow, own and prepare.

You will need:

2 cups Wild Lettuce

Cheese cloth / Dark container

Directions:

(If freshly grown, grind up in a blender with just enough water to cover lettuce).

-In a pot or crock pot, low cook (not boil) 2 cups of Wild Lettuce.

-Add just enough water to cover plant matter

-Low cook for 30 mins. Be sure not to boil or you can destroy the medicine.

-Remove from stove and drain out pain medicine through cheese cloth.

-Clean pot then add strained medicine juice back to pot.

-Simmer (not boil), black liquid until most of the water has evaporated and it becomes a dark gel. Be careful not to boil. Stir often. May take several hours for water to evaporate.

-Once it becomes black gel, add it to dark jar and store in cool, dark, place.

-Wild Lettuce dosing is different for each person. Take 1/4 teaspoon every 45 mins to gauge how much is necessary.

Recipe 15: Wild Lettuce Capsules

You will need:

Coffee grinder

Dehydrator

Capsule machine

Directions:

-Take Lettuce Gel from previous recipe and put into a dehydrator.

-Smooth out as thin as possible before putting into the dehydrator.

-Set dehydrator to 114-118 degrees, dehydrate until dry.

-Break apart Lettuce sheet.

-Put into coffee grinder to powder. Then pill powder with capsule machine.

-Not needed but always good to store in cool dry place.

-Start with 1 pill every 45 mins., until pain subsides to gauge tolerance and how much is needed.

Recipe 16: MSM Aloe Pain Gel

You will need:

In a Mason Jar combine:

3 tbsp. Pure MSM Powder

1/2 cup Aloe Gel

10 drops Kopaebo Essential Oil

5 drops Lavender Essential Oil

5 drops Peppermint Essential Oil

-Close jar and shake well before each use.

-Apply to pain area as needed.

-Store in cool dark place.

Recipe 17: Gout Relief

You will need:

1 Liter of black cherry juice

1 Liter of fresh juiced celery

4 bananas

2- 1-liter sized containers.

Directions:

-In each liter container combine ½ liter of juiced celery and ½ liter of cherry juice.

-Drink 1 liter of this mix each day.

*Warning: This recipe will cause gas and diarrhea. The juice is expelling toxins and uric acid from the body which is the cause of the gout pain.

Consume 1 banana every 30 mins. when your stomach has been completely cleaned out, usually by the 4th hour. Taking bananas will close stomach and stop the diarrhea.

If gout pain persists, repeat remedy the next day also. Gout pain should be gone by or before 3rd day.

Other things that help with Gout pain management

-Consuming high doses of Vitamin C, help with Gout pain.

1,000mg Emergen C packs every 3 hours is suggested.

-Consuming fruits like cherries, pineapples, apples, bananas and strawberries help in curing gout pain.

-Soaking the area in a bucket of warm water with:

1/2 cup Charcoal Powder or

1/4 cup of Cayanne Pepper

-Rubbing the area with Wintergreen Oil 2-3 times per day, can also relieve the pain.

-Soaking the area in an ice bath for 20 mins can also reduce inflammation.

-Soak affected area in Rosemary Essential Oil and Epson Salt bath, also helps the pain.

Find out what is causing Gout and STOP CONSUMING IT!

Glossary

1)What is a carrier Oil?

Any oil used in an infusion.

2)What is an infusion?

An infusion is when you extract and bind any type of plant matter with a carrier oil.

3)How to use a crock-pot to make a quick oil infusion.

<u>You will need:</u>

-A Crock-pot and lid

-Mason Jar that fits in the crock pot

-Baking bags

-Rubber band

-Your choice of carrier oil

-Your choice of plant matter

<u>Directions:</u>

-Fill crock-pot ¾ full of water

-Cut a piece of the baking bag to fit the top of the Mason Jar. Make sure you cut a piece big enough to be secured by the rubber band.

-Fill Mason Jar 3/4 full of plant matter.

-Cover plant matter with carrier oil.

-Cover jar with pre-cut baking bag, and tightly secure with rubber band.

-Place jar in crock-pot.

-Add water to crock-pot, water should rise up ¾ of the height of the jar, but not submerge the jar.

-Cover crock-pot with lid. Plug in and turn on lowest setting. Usually that's "warm".

-Let the infusion cook overnight or for at least 12 hours. It should be done in the morning. Strain the matter CAUTIOUSLY, for it will be hot. Label and put it in a dark jar away from the sunlight.

Thank you for your purchase. This is

the 1st volume in a series of "Plant to medicine" natural remedy recipe books. Please remember that when it comes to organic medicine, not all remedies work for everyone the same. Everyone's health, environment, and living condition is different. So be safe, careful, and find what works for your situation. Healing is all around us, planted in the Garden God gave us. If you feed your body what it needs to heal itself, it will heal. Be well, Be Blessed, and Remember....

"Plants are medicine"

We will have many more recipe books. The upcoming volumes will list recipes for fixing Eyes, Cancer, Mental health issues, and much much more! There are plants to help fix everything.

For free recipes and videos follow me on

www.instagram.com/papabearpantry

Or

facebook@Papabear'sPantry@Papabear992